100 Day Tear-Off Diet Countdown Calendar

Transcripture International

100 Day Tear-Off Diet Countdown Calendar

ISBN-13: 978-1922217561

Published by Transcripture International.

For inquiries and bulk orders please visit http://www.buycountdowncalendar.com/

20140101190608-100-P

How to Use This Calendar

Please seek medical advice before starting any diet or exercise plan.

Step 1: Decide How to Hang

This calendar is best viewed when hung on a wall.

Below are some suggested hanging methods:

1) Make holes through the two outermost guide marks on the cover near the binding and hang the calendar with string.

2) Make a hole through the middle guide mark on the cover and hang on a nail or screw.

3) Push thumb tacks through the back cover to attach the calendar to a pin board

4) Glue the back cover to a larger piece of cardboard that can be attached to or hung on a wall.

Step 2: Prepare for Hanging

Remove the front cover and the first two pages, including this page, to expose the first day.

The last page of this calendar is blank so you can remove the last printed page and display something else such as a special message or photograph instead if you wish.

Step 3: Start the Countdown!

Hang the calendar as desired then, as each day passes, remove one page by tearing or cutting along the guideline.

100

DAYS LEFT

99

DAYS LEFT

98

DAYS LEFT

97

DAYS LEFT

96

DAYS LEFT

95

DAYS LEFT

94

DAYS LEFT

93

DAYS LEFT

92

DAYS LEFT

19 DAYS LEFT

90

DAYS LEFT

98

DAYS LEFT

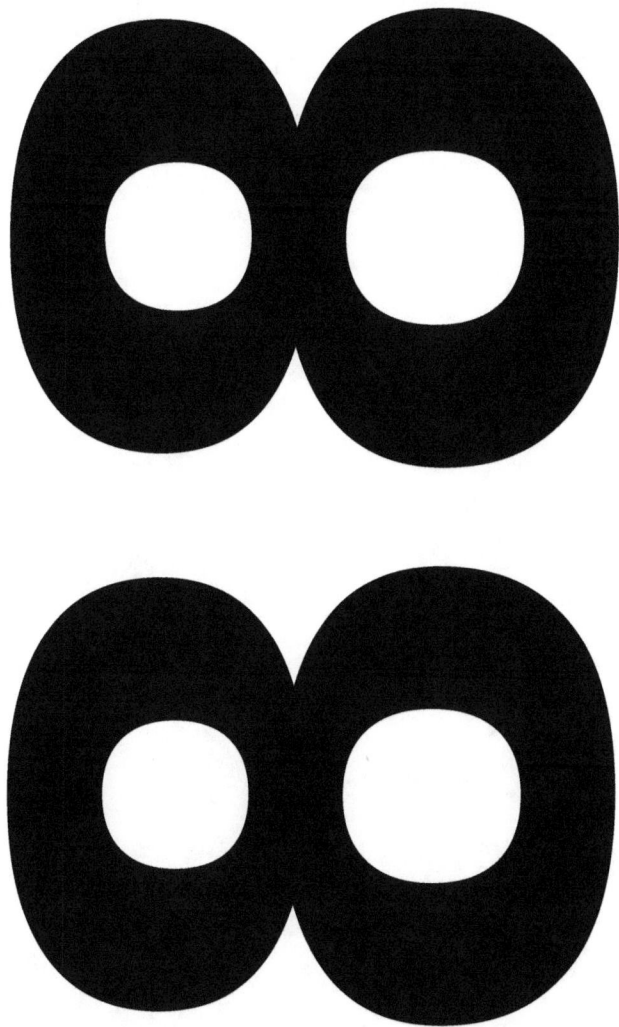

88

DAYS LEFT

78

DAYS LEFT

68

DAYS LEFT

58

DAYS LEFT

48

DAYS LEFT

38 DAYS LEFT

28

DAYS LEFT

18

DAYS LEFT

80

DAYS LEFT

79

DAYS LEFT

78

DAYS LEFT

7

DAYS LEFT

76

DAYS LEFT

157

DAYS LEFT

74

DAYS LEFT

73

DAYS LEFT

21

DAYS LEFT

17 DAYS LEFT

70

DAYS LEFT

69

DAYS LEFT

60

DAYS LEFT

76

DAYS LEFT

60

DAYS LEFT

5 6 5

DAYS LEFT

64 DAYS LEFT

3

60

DAYS LEFT

26

DAYS LEFT

16 DAYS LEFT

60

DAYS LEFT

95

DAYS LEFT

8

50

DAYS LEFT

75

DAYS LEFT

56

DAYS LEFT

55

DAYS LEFT

54

DAYS LEFT

35 DAYS LEFT

252

DAYS LEFT

15 DAYS LEFT

50

DAYS LEFT

49

DAYS LEFT

48

DAYS LEFT

74

DAYS LEFT

46

DAYS LEFT

45

DAYS LEFT

44

DAYS LEFT

34

DAYS LEFT

24

DAYS LEFT

14 DAYS LEFT

40

DAYS LEFT

39

DAYS LEFT

30

DAYS LEFT

73

DAYS LEFT

30 DAYS LEFT

135

DAYS LEFT

34

DAYS LEFT

3

3

DAYS LEFT

23

DAYS LEFT

13

DAYS LEFT

30

DAYS LEFT

29

DAYS LEFT

82

DAYS LEFT

72

DAYS LEFT

26

DAYS LEFT

52

DAYS LEFT

24

DAYS LEFT

32

DAYS LEFT

22

DAYS LEFT

12 DAYS LEFT

02

DAYS LEFT

19

DAYS LEFT

8

1

DAYS LEFT

1 DAYS LEFT

16

DAYS LEFT

15

DAYS LEFT

14

DAYS LEFT

3 DAYS LEFT

21

DAYS LEFT

11

DAYS LEFT

10

DAYS LEFT

9

DAYS LEFT

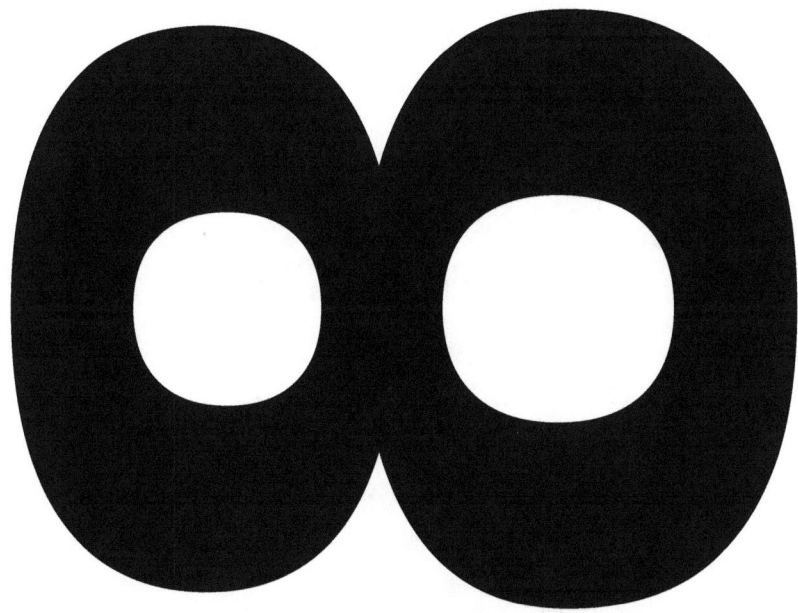

8 DAYS LEFT

1 DAYS LEFT

6 DAYS LEFT

5

DAYS LEFT

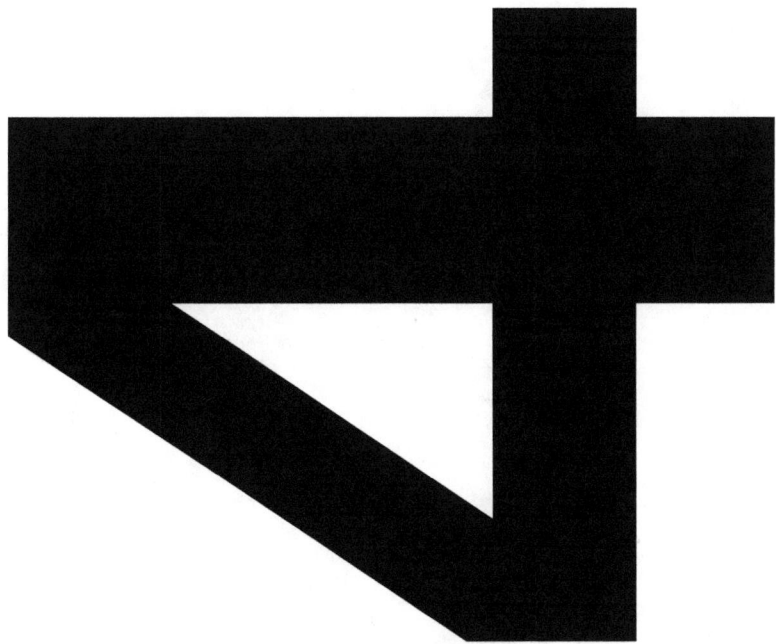

4

DAYS LEFT

3

DAYS LEFT

2 DAYS LEFT

1 DAY LEFT

O

DAYS LEFT